Zero Point Outdoor Gas Griddle Recipes For Weight Loss

Unlock the Secrets to Delicious and Tasty Zero Point Gas Griddle Recipes for Lasting Weight Loss Success and a Healthier You.

CLARE A. DEEN

Copyright Page

TABLE OF CONTENTS

UNDERSTANDING THE CONCEPT OF ZERO POINT FOOD

Zero Point foods is designed to support a balanced and sustainable approach to healthy eating, focusing on nutrient-dense foods while allowing for flexibility and enjoyment in food choices. Here's a breakdown of the concept and how it works:

1. **Nutrient-rich foods**: Zero Point foods typically include fruits, vegetables, lean proteins, and some whole grains. These foods are chosen because they tend to be lower in calories while providing essential nutrients like vitamins, minerals, fiber, and protein.

- **Freedom to eat**: When a food is designated as a Zero Point food, it means you can eat it without having to track or count its SmartPoints value. This provides a sense of freedom and flexibility in meal planning and allows you to focus on eating nutritious foods that help you feel satisfied and energized.

- **Encourages healthy choices**: By emphasizing Zero Point foods, the program encourages participants to base their meals around these healthier options.

- This can help improve overall dietary patterns by increasing intake of fruits, vegetables, and lean proteins, which are associated with numerous health benefits, including weight management, improved digestion, and reduced risk of chronic diseases.

- **Portion control:** While Zero Point foods are free to eat, portion control is still important. Eating unlimited quantities of even healthy foods can lead to overconsumption of calories, which may hinder weight loss or maintenance goals. The program encourages mindful eating and listening to hunger and fullness cues to help regulate portion sizes.

- **Flexibility:** Although Zero Point foods are encouraged, the program also allows for flexibility and moderation. Participants still have a daily Smart Points budget that can be used for foods that are not Zero Point, such as treats or higher-calorie items. This flexibility makes the program sustainable and adaptable to individual preferences and lifestyles.

HOW ZERO POINT FOODS CONTRIBUTE TO A HEALTHY LIFESTYLE

Zero-point foods contribute to a healthy lifestyle by providing essential nutrients, supporting weight management, reducing the risk of chronic diseases, boosting immune function, promoting healthy aging, improving mood and mental health, increasing energy levels, supporting environmental sustainability, and being budget-friendly.

- **Nutrient Density:** Many zero-point foods are rich in essential nutrients such as vitamins, minerals, and antioxidants.

- **Calorie Control:** Since zero-point foods are low in calories, they can help with calorie control and weight management. They allow you to fill up on nutritious options without consuming excessive calories, making it easier to maintain a healthy weight.

- **Hydration:** Many zero-point foods, especially fruits and vegetables, have high water content, which contributes to hydration.

- **Blood Sugar Control:** Foods like non-starchy vegetables and lean proteins have minimal impact on blood sugar levels, which is beneficial for individuals with diabetes or those looking to stabilize their blood sugar levels.

- **Heart Health:** Many zero-point foods, such as fruits, vegetables, and lean proteins, are beneficial for heart health due to their low saturated fat and cholesterol content.
- **Digestive Health:** The fiber found in many zero-point foods supports digestive health by promoting regular bowel movements and preventing constipation.
- **Reduced Risk of Chronic Diseases:** A diet rich in zero-point foods, particularly fruits and vegetables, has been linked to a reduced risk of chronic diseases such as certain cancers, cardiovascular disease, and diabetes.
- **Improved Immune Function:** Many zero-point foods, especially fruits and vegetables, are rich in vitamins A, C, and E, as well as other nutrients that support immune function.

STEPS TO EFFECTIVELY USE A GAS GRIDDLE

- **Preheat the Griddle:** Before you start cooking, preheat the griddle for about 10-15 minutes. This allows the cooking surface to reach the desired temperature and ensures even cooking.

- **Season the Griddle (if needed):** Some griddles may require seasoning before use, especially if they are made of cast iron. Follow the manufacturer's instructions for seasoning if necessary.

- **Adjust the Temperature:** Gas griddles typically have temperature controls that allow you to adjust the heat. Adjust the temperature according to the recipe you're following or the type of food you're cooking. For example, you may need higher heat for searing meats and lower heat for cooking delicate foods like pancakes.

- **Oil the Griddle:** Before adding food, lightly oil the griddle surface to prevent sticking. You can use a high-heat oil like vegetable oil or canola oil. Spread the oil evenly across the surface using a brush or paper towel.

- **Cooking:** Place the food on the griddle once it's hot and oiled. Cook the food according to your recipe, flipping it as needed for even cooking. Avoid overcrowding the griddle, as this can lower the temperature and result in uneven cooking.

- **Cleaning:** After you're done cooking, allow the griddle to cool down completely. Use a scraper or spatula to remove any food residue from the surface. For tougher residue, you can use warm soapy water and a sponge to clean the griddle. Avoid using abrasive cleaners or metal utensils that can scratch the surface.

- **Maintenance:** Regularly clean and maintain your gas griddle to ensure its longevity and performance. Follow the manufacturer's instructions for proper care and storage.

SHOPPING FOR ZERO POINT FOODS

Shopping for zero point foods typically involves selecting foods that are low in calories and high in nutrients, as they are designated as "zero points" on certain weight loss programs. Here's a list of common zero point foods:

- **Fruits:** *Apples, Bananas, Berries (strawberries, blueberries, raspberries, blackberries), Oranges, Grapefruit, Peaches, Pears, Plums, Kiwi, Melons (watermelon, cantaloupe, honeydew), Grapes, Pineapple, Mango, Cherries etc.*

- **Vegetables:** *Spinach, Kale, Lettuce (all varieties), Arugula, Swiss chard, Collard greens, Mustard greens, Turnip greens, Beet greens, Broccoli, Cauliflower, Carrots, Bell peppers (all colors), Cucumbers, Tomatoes, Celery, Radishes, Green beans, Snap peas, Asparagus, Zucchini, Summer squash, Eggplant, Mushrooms, Onions, Garlic, Leeks, Scallions, Brussels sprouts, Cabbage (green, red, Napa), Spaghetti squash, Butternut squash, Acorn squash, Pumpkin*

- **Lean proteins:** *Skinless chicken breast, turkey breast, tofu, fish (such as salmon or cod), shellfish (like shrimp or crab), eggs, plain Greek yogurt (non-fat), cottage cheese (non-fat), beans, lentils, etc.*

- **Whole grains:** *Quinoa, brown rice, oats, barley, whole wheat pasta, etc.*

- **Non-starchy vegetables:** *Asparagus, cauliflower, zucchini, cabbage, kale, Brussels sprouts, etc.*

- **Condiments and seasonings:** *Herbs, spices, vinegar, mustard, hot sauce, salsa, Lemon juice, Lime juice, Pickles (dill, gherkins, etc.), Capers, Unsweetened almond milk, Unsweetened coconut milk, Unsweetened soy milk etc.*

When shopping for zero point foods, focus on fresh produce, lean proteins, and whole grains. Avoid processed foods and those high in added sugars and fats. It's also essential to read labels carefully, as some foods may seem healthy but can contain hidden sugars or unhealthy fats. Buying in bulk and planning meals ahead of time can help you incorporate these zero point foods into your diet effectively.

WHAT TO AVOID WHEN SHOPPING FOR ZERO POINT FOODS

When shopping for Zero Point Foods, which are often associated with weight loss and healthy eating plans, it's essential to be mindful of a few key considerations to ensure you're making the healthiest choices possible. Here are some things to avoid:

- **Processed Foods**: While some processed foods may still be considered Zero Point Foods due to their low-calorie content, they may lack essential nutrients and contain additives, preservatives, and excessive sodium or sugar.
- **Added Sugars:** Even if a food is listed as a Zero Point Food, it's crucial to check the label for added sugars. High sugar intake can lead to various health issues, including weight gain, diabetes, and heart disease.
- **Highly Caloric Foods:** While Zero Point Foods are meant to be low in calories, some naturally calorie-dense foods, like nuts and avocados, are not included in this category. While they are healthy in moderation, consuming them excessively could hinder weight loss efforts.

- **Overindulgence:** Just because a food is labeled as Zero Points doesn't mean you should consume unlimited quantities of it. Portion control is still important for overall health and weight management.
- **Ignoring All Other Nutritional Information:** While a food may be Zero Points, it's essential to consider its overall nutritional value. For example, a food may be low in calories but high in unhealthy fats or lacking in essential vitamins and minerals.

GRILLED LEMON PEPPER SHRIMP SKEWERS

PREP
10 Mins

COOK
8 Mins

YIELDS
4 Servings

Marinating Time: 30 Mins

INGREDIENTS

- 1 pound large shrimp, peeled and deveined
- 2 lemons, juiced and zested
- 2 teaspoons olive oil
- 2 teaspoons freshly ground black pepper
- 1 teaspoon garlic powder
- 1 teaspoon onion powder
- Salt to taste
- Skewers, soaked in water if wooden

DIRECTIONS

- In a bowl, combine the shrimp, lemon juice, lemon zest, olive oil, black pepper, garlic powder, onion powder, and salt. Toss to coat the shrimp evenly. Let it marinate for at least 30 minutes in the refrigerator.
- Preheat your grill to medium-high heat.
- Thread the marinated shrimp onto skewers, dividing them evenly.
- Place the skewers on the preheated grill. Grill for 2-3 minutes per side, or until the shrimp are pink and opaque.
- Once grilled, remove the skewers from the grill and serve immediately.

NUTRITIONAL FACTS (PER SERVING)

- Calories: 120kcal
- Protein: 22g
- Fat: 2g
- Carbohydrates: 4g
- Fiber: 1g
- Sugar: 1g

GRIDDLED GREEK CHICKEN GYROS

PREP
40 Mins

COOK
12 Mins

YIELDS
4 Servings

Prep Time includes marinating time

INGREDIENTS

- 1 lb (450g) boneless, skinless chicken breasts, thinly sliced
- 1 tablespoon olive oil
- 2 cloves garlic, minced
- 1 teaspoon dried oregano
- 1 teaspoon dried thyme
- 1 teaspoon dried rosemary
- Salt and pepper to taste
- Juice of 1 lemon
- 4 whole wheat pitas
- Tzatziki sauce (store-bought or homemade)
- Sliced tomatoes, onions, and lettuce for garnish

DIRECTIONS

- In a large bowl, combine olive oil, minced garlic, dried oregano, thyme, rosemary, salt, pepper, and lemon juice. Add sliced chicken breasts to the bowl and toss until evenly coated. Let marinate for at least 30 minutes in the refrigerator.
- Heat a griddle or large skillet over medium-high heat. Once hot, add the marinated chicken slices and cook for 5-6 minutes per side, or until cooked through and nicely browned. Remove from heat and set aside.
- While the chicken is cooking, warm the whole wheat pitas on the griddle for about 1 minute on each side, or until lightly toasted.

NUTRITIONAL FACTS (PER SERVING)

- Calories: 350kcal
- Protein: 30g
- Carbohydrates: 30g
- Fat: 12g
- Fiber: 6g
- Sugar: 3g

DIRECTIONS

- To assemble the gyros, spread a generous amount of tzatziki sauce on each warm pita. Top with slices of cooked chicken, sliced tomatoes, onions, and lettuce.
- Serve immediately and enjoy!

BBQ CHICKEN BREAST WITH GRILLED VEGETABLES

 **Prep Time**
15 Mins

Cook Time
20 Mins

 **Yields**
4 Servings

INGREDIENTS

- 4 boneless, skinless chicken breasts
- 1 cup of your favorite sugar-free BBQ sauce
- 2 medium zucchinis, sliced
- 2 bell peppers (any color), sliced
- 1 large red onion, sliced
- 2 tablespoons olive oil
- Salt and pepper to taste
- Optional: additional seasoning for chicken (e.g., garlic powder, paprika)

DIRECTIONS

- Preheat your grill to medium-high heat.
- Season chicken breasts with salt, pepper, and any additional seasoning you prefer.
- Brush the chicken breasts with BBQ sauce on both sides.
- In a large bowl, toss sliced zucchinis, bell peppers, and red onion with olive oil, salt, and pepper.
- Place the chicken breasts on the grill and cook for about 6-7 minutes on each side, or until cooked through with nice grill marks.
- While the chicken is cooking, place the vegetables on the grill and cook for about 5-6 minutes, or until tender and slightly charred, flipping halfway through.

NUTRITIONAL FACTS (PER SERVING)

- Calories: 300kcal
- Protein: 30g
- Carbohydrates: 20g
- Fat: 10g
- Fiber: 5g

DIRECTIONS

- Once the chicken and vegetables are cooked, remove them from the grill.
- Serve the BBQ chicken breasts alongside the grilled vegetables.

TERIYAKI SALMON WITH GRILLED PINEAPPLE

PREP
10 Mins

COOK
10 Mins

YIELDS
4 Servings

Marinating time: 2 hrs

INGREDIENTS

- 4 salmon fillets
- 1 cup teriyaki sauce (look for a low-sodium or reduced-sugar option if you're following WW)
- 1 tablespoon olive oil
- 1 teaspoon minced garlic
- 1 teaspoon minced ginger
- 1 pineapple, peeled and sliced into rings
- Salt and pepper to taste
- Chopped green onions and sesame seeds for garnish (optional)

DIRECTIONS

- In a bowl, mix together the teriyaki sauce, olive oil, minced garlic, and minced ginger.
- Place the salmon fillets in a shallow dish or a resealable plastic bag, and pour the teriyaki marinade over them. Make sure the salmon is well coated. Marinate in the refrigerator for at least 30 minutes, or up to 2 hours.
- Preheat your grill to medium-high heat.
- Remove the salmon from the marinade and discard any excess marinade.
- Season the salmon with salt and pepper to taste.
- Place the salmon fillets on the grill, skin-side down,

NUTRITIONAL FACTS (PER SERVING)

- Calories: 300kcal
- Protein: 25g
- Fat: 12g
- Carbohydrates: 25g
- Fiber: 2g
- Sugar: 20g

DIRECTIONS

- and cook for 4-5 minutes per side, or until the salmon is cooked through and easily flakes with a fork.
- While the salmon is cooking, grill the pineapple rings for 2-3 minutes per side, until they have grill marks and are heated through.
- Serve the grilled salmon with the grilled pineapple slices on the side. Garnish with chopped green onions and sesame seeds if desired.

TURKEY BURGER SLIDERS WITH GRILLED ONIONS

PREP
15 Mins

COOK
15 Mins

YIELDS
8 Servings

INGREDIENTS

- 1 pound ground turkey breast
- 1/4 cup finely chopped onion
- 1 clove garlic, minced
- 1 teaspoon Worcestershire sauce
- 1/2 teaspoon salt
- 1/4 teaspoon black pepper
- 1 large onion, sliced into rings for grilling
- Slider buns (whole wheat or low-calorie, if preferred)
- Lettuce leaves (optional)
- Tomato slices (optional)

DIRECTIONS

- Preheat your grill or grill pan to medium-high heat.
- In a mixing bowl, combine the ground turkey, finely chopped onion, minced garlic, Worcestershire sauce, salt, and black pepper. Mix well until all ingredients are evenly distributed.
- Form the turkey mixture into small patties, about the size of slider buns. Make an indentation in the center of each patty with your thumb to prevent them from puffing up while cooking.
- Place the turkey patties on the preheated grill and cook for about 4-5 minutes on each side, or until they are cooked through and no longer pink in the center.

NUTRITIONAL FACTS (PER SERVING)

- Calories: 150kcal
- Total Fat: 5g
- Saturated Fat: 1g
- Cholesterol: 35mg
- Sodium: 250mg
- Carbohydrates: 13g
- Dietary Fiber: 2g
- Sugars: 2g
- Protein: 13g

DIRECTIONS

- While the turkey patties are cooking, grill the sliced onions until they are caramelized and tender, about 5-7 minutes per side.
- Toast the slider buns on the grill for about 1-2 minutes, until they are lightly browned.
- Assemble the sliders by placing a turkey patty on the bottom half of each bun, then top with grilled onions, lettuce leaves, and tomato slices if desired. Place the top half of the bun over the toppings to complete the sliders.
- Serve immediately and enjoy!

GRIDDLED VEGETABLE STIR-FRY

PREP
10 Mins

COOK
15 Mins

YIELDS
4 Servings

INGREDIENTS

- Assorted zero-point vegetables such as bell peppers, mushrooms, zucchini, broccoli, onions, etc.
- Low-sodium soy sauce or tamari
- Minced garlic
- Minced ginger
- Optional: sliced chicken breast or tofu for added protein (points would need to be calculated for these)

DIRECTIONS

- Wash and chop all the vegetables into bite-sized pieces.
- Preheat a griddle or large skillet over medium-high heat.
- If using chicken breast or tofu, cook them first until they're browned and cooked through. Remove from the griddle and set aside.
- Add a splash of water or low-sodium broth to the griddle to prevent sticking.
- Add minced garlic and ginger to the griddle and cook for about 30 seconds until fragrant.
- Add the chopped vegetables to the griddle. Cook, stirring occasionally, until they are tender-crisp, about 8-10 minutes.

NUTRITIONAL FACTS (PER SERVING)

- Calories: 50kcal
- Total Fat: 0.5g
- Carbohydrates: 10g
- Dietary Fiber: 3g
- Sugars: 4g
- Protein: 3g

DIRECTIONS

- If using, add the cooked chicken breast or tofu back to the griddle and toss with the vegetables.
- Pour low-sodium soy sauce or tamari over the stir-fry and toss to combine.
- Cook for another 1-2 minutes to let the flavors meld.
- Remove from heat and serve hot. Enjoy your zero-point griddled vegetable stir-fry!

KOREAN BBQ BEEF BULGOGI

 **Prep Time**
2 Mins

Cook Time
4 Mins

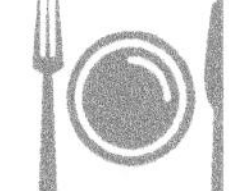 **Yields**
4 Servings

INGREDIENTS

- 1 lb thinly sliced beef (such as ribeye or sirloin)
- 1/2 cup soy sauce (low sodium if preferred)
- 1/4 cup brown sugar or sweetener of choice
- 4 cloves garlic, minced
- 1 small onion, thinly sliced
- 2 green onions, chopped
- 1 tablespoon sesame oil
- 1 tablespoon sesame seeds
- 1/2 teaspoon black pepper
- Optional: sliced mushrooms, bell peppers, or other vegetables

DIRECTIONS

Preparation:

- In a bowl, mix together soy sauce, brown sugar, minced garlic, sliced onion, chopped green onions, sesame oil, sesame seeds, and black pepper to create the marinade.
- Place the thinly sliced beef in a large resealable plastic bag or shallow dish.
- Pour the marinade over the beef, making sure it's evenly coated. Seal the bag or cover the dish, then refrigerate for at least 1 hour, or preferably overnight to allow the flavors to meld.

Cooking Instructions:

- Heat a grill pan or skillet over medium-high heat.

NUTRITIONAL FACTS (PER SERVING)

- Calories: 300kcal
- Protein: 25g
- Fat: 15g
- Carbohydrates: 15g
- Fiber: 2g
- Sodium: 900mg

DIRECTIONS

- Once hot, add the marinated beef slices in a single layer, working in batches if necessary to avoid overcrowding the pan.
- Cook for about 2-3 minutes on each side, or until the beef is cooked through and caramelized on the edges.
- Optional: While cooking the beef, you can also grill or sauté the optional vegetables until tender.

Serving:

- Serve the cooked beef bulgogi hot, garnished with additional chopped green onions and sesame seeds if desired.
- You can serve it over steamed rice, lettuce leaves for wrapping (ssam), or with a side of kimchi or pickled vegetables.

GRILLED PORTOBELLO MUSHROOM "STEAKS"

PREP
10 Mins

COOK
10 Mins

YIELDS
4 Servings

INGREDIENTS

- 4 large Portobello mushrooms
- 2 tablespoons balsamic vinegar
- 2 tablespoons low-sodium soy sauce
- 2 cloves garlic, minced
- 1 teaspoon dried thyme
- Salt and pepper to taste
- Optional: your choice of herbs or spices for added flavor

DIRECTIONS

- Clean the Portobello mushrooms by wiping them with a damp cloth. Remove the stems and any gills from the underside of the mushrooms.
- In a small bowl, whisk together the balsamic vinegar, soy sauce, minced garlic, dried thyme, salt, and pepper.
- Place the cleaned mushrooms in a shallow dish or large resealable plastic bag. Pour the marinade over the mushrooms, making sure they are well coated. Marinate for at least 30 minutes, turning the mushrooms occasionally to ensure they are evenly coated.
- Preheat your grill to medium-high heat. Lightly oil the grill grates to prevent sticking.

NUTRITIONAL FACTS
(PER SERVING)

- Calories: 35kcal
- Total Fat: 0.5g
- Saturated Fat: 0g
- Cholesterol: 0mg
- Sodium: 175mg
- Carbohydrates: 5g
- Dietary Fiber: 1g
- Sugars: 2g
- Protein: 3g

DIRECTIONS

- Remove the mushrooms from the marinade, shaking off any excess liquid. Reserve the marinade for basting.
- Place the mushrooms on the grill, gill side down. Grill for 4-5 minutes on each side, or until the mushrooms are tender and slightly charred, basting occasionally with the reserved marinade.
- Once cooked, remove the mushrooms from the grill and serve hot. You can garnish with additional herbs or spices if desired.

GRILLED LEMON HERB SWORDFISH

PREP
10 Mins

COOK
10 Mins

YIELDS
4 Servings

INGREDIENTS

- 4 swordfish steaks (about 6 ounces each)
- 2 tablespoons olive oil
- 2 cloves garlic, minced
- Zest of 1 lemon
- Juice of 1 lemon
- 2 tablespoons fresh chopped parsley
- Salt and pepper to taste

DIRECTIONS

- Preheat your grill to medium-high heat.
- In a small bowl, mix together the olive oil, minced garlic, lemon zest, lemon juice, chopped parsley, salt, and pepper.
- Brush both sides of the swordfish steaks with the lemon herb mixture.
- Place the swordfish steaks on the preheated grill and cook for about 4-5 minutes per side, or until the fish is cooked through and easily flakes with a fork.
- Remove the swordfish from the grill and serve immediately.

NUTRITIONAL FACTS (PER SERVING)

- Calories: 280kcal
- Total Fat: 14g
- Saturated Fat: 2g
- Cholesterol: 80mg
- Sodium: 120mg
- Carbohydrates: 1g
- Dietary Fiber: 0g
- Sugars: 0g
- Protein: 35g

CAJUN GRILLED CATFISH FILLETS

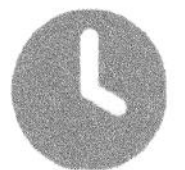 **Prep Time**
10 Mins

Cook Time
10 Mins

 **Yields**
4 Servings

INGREDIENTS

- 4 catfish fillets (about 6 ounces each)
- 2 teaspoons paprika
- 1 teaspoon garlic powder
- 1 teaspoon onion powder
- 1 teaspoon dried thyme
- 1 teaspoon dried oregano
- 1/2 teaspoon cayenne pepper (adjust to taste)
- 1/2 teaspoon black pepper
- 1/2 teaspoon salt
- Cooking spray

DIRECTIONS

- In a small bowl, mix together paprika, garlic powder, onion powder, thyme, oregano, cayenne pepper, black pepper, and salt to create the Cajun seasoning.
- Pat dry the catfish fillets with paper towels.
- Rub the Cajun seasoning evenly over both sides of the catfish fillets.
- Preheat grill to medium-high heat.
- Spray the grill grates lightly with cooking spray to prevent sticking.
- Place the seasoned catfish fillets on the grill and cook for about 4-5 minutes per side, or until the fish is opaque and easily flakes with a fork.
- Remove the catfish fillets from the grill and serve immediately.

NUTRITIONAL FACTS
(PER SERVING)

- Calories: 160kcal
- Total Fat: 2g
- Saturated Fat: 0.5g
- Cholesterol: 90mg
- Sodium: 380mg
- Carbohydrates: 2g
- Dietary Fiber: 1g
- Sugars: 0g
- Protein: 32g

HONEY MUSTARD GLAZED GRILLED PORK CHOPS

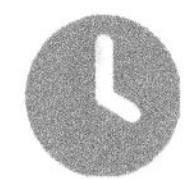 **Prep Time**
35 Mins

Cook Time
14 Mins

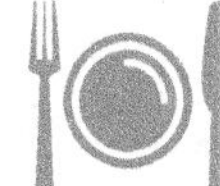 **Yields**
4 Servings

INGREDIENTS

- 4 boneless pork chops
- ¼ cup Dijon mustard
- 2 tablespoons honey
- 1 tablespoon olive oil
- 2 cloves garlic, minced
- Salt and pepper to taste
- Optional: chopped fresh parsley for garnish

DIRECTIONS

- In a small bowl, mix together the Dijon mustard, honey, olive oil, minced garlic, salt, and pepper to create the glaze.
- Place the pork chops in a shallow dish or resealable plastic bag and pour half of the glaze over them. Reserve the other half of the glaze for later.
- Allow the pork chops to marinate in the refrigerator for at least 30 minutes, or up to 4 hours if time allows.
- Preheat your grill to medium-high heat.
- Remove the pork chops from the marinade and discard any excess marinade.
- Grill the pork chops for 5-7 minutes per side,

NUTRITIONAL FACTS (PER SERVING)

- Calories: 250kcal
- Total Fat: 10g
- Saturated Fat: 2g
- Cholesterol: 70mg
- Sodium: 300mg
- Carbohydrates: 10g
- Dietary Fiber: 0g
- Sugars: 8g
- Protein: 30g

DIRECTIONS

- or until they reach an internal temperature of 145°F (63°C), brushing with the reserved glaze during the last few minutes of cooking.
- Once cooked through, remove the pork chops from the grill and let them rest for a few minutes before serving.
- Garnish with chopped fresh parsley if desired, and serve hot.

GRILLED VEGETABLE SALAD

 **Prep Time**
15 Mins

Cook Time
20 Mins

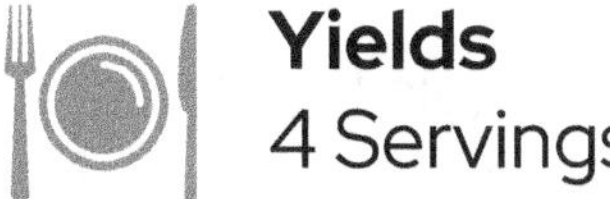 **Yields**
4 Servings

INGREDIENTS

- Assorted vegetables (such as bell peppers, zucchini, eggplant, onions, mushrooms)
- Salt and pepper to taste
- Fresh herbs (such as parsley, basil, or thyme)
- Balsamic vinegar or lemon juice for dressing

DIRECTIONS

- Wash and chop the vegetables into bite-sized pieces.
- Preheat your grill to medium-high heat.
- Season the vegetables with salt, pepper, and any desired herbs.
- Grill the vegetables until they are tender and have grill marks, about 5-10 minutes per side depending on the vegetable.
- Remove the vegetables from the grill and let them cool slightly.
- Toss the grilled vegetables with balsamic vinegar or lemon juice for dressing.
- Serve warm or at room temperature.

NUTRITIONAL FACTS (PER SERVING)

- Calories: 160kcal
- Protein: 25g
- Fat: 4g
- Carbohydrates: 7g
- Fiber: 2g

STRAWBERRY MINT SMOOTHIE

 **Prep Time**
5 Mins

Cook Time
0 Mins

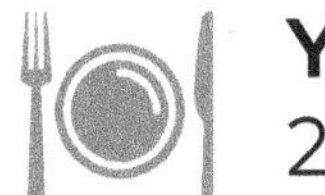 **Yields**
2 Servings

INGREDIENTS

- 1 cup fresh or frozen strawberries (zero points)
- 1/2 medium banana, sliced (zero points)
- 1/2 cup fat-free Greek yogurt (zero points)
- 1/2 cup unsweetened almond milk (zero points)
- 1-2 tablespoons fresh mint leaves, to taste (zero points)
- Ice cubes (optional)

DIRECTIONS

- Place strawberries, banana slices, Greek yogurt, almond milk, and fresh mint leaves in a blender.
- Blend until smooth. If you prefer a thicker consistency, you can add ice cubes and blend again.
- Pour the smoothie into a glass and garnish with additional mint leaves if desired.
- Enjoy your refreshing Zero Point WW Strawberry Mint Smoothie guilt-free!

NUTRITIONAL FACTS
(PER SERVING)

- Calories: 200kcal
- Protein: 15g
- Carbohydrates: 40g
- Fat: 2g
- Fiber: 8g
- Sugar: 20g

GRIDDLED TOFU VEGGIE SKEWERS

 **Prep Time**
40 Mins

Cook Time
10 Mins

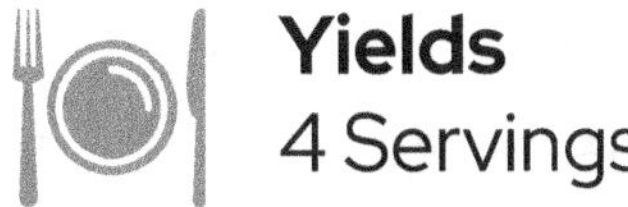 **Yields**
4 Servings

INGREDIENTS

- 1 block extra firm tofu, pressed and cut into cubes
- 1 zucchini, sliced into rounds
- 1 bell pepper, cut into chunks
- 1 red onion, cut into chunks
- Cherry tomatoes
- Wooden skewers, soaked in water for at least 30 minutes

Marinade:

- 2 tablespoons soy sauce (low-sodium if desired)
- 1 tablespoon rice vinegar
- 1 tablespoon maple syrup
- 1 teaspoon minced garlic
- 1 teaspoon grated ginger
- 1 teaspoon sesame oil
- Salt and pepper to taste

DIRECTIONS

- In a small bowl, whisk together all marinade ingredients.
- Place tofu cubes in a shallow dish or resealable bag and pour marinade over tofu. Allow to marinate for at least 30 minutes, or overnight for best flavor.
- Preheat griddle pan or grill over medium-high heat.
- Thread marinated tofu cubes, zucchini slices, bell pepper chunks, red onion chunks, and cherry tomatoes onto soaked wooden skewers, alternating the vegetables and tofu.
- Place skewers on the preheated griddle pan or grill and cook for 8-10 minutes,

NUTRITIONAL FACTS (PER SERVING)

- Calories: 150kcal
- Total Fat: 6g
- Saturated Fat: 1g
- Trans Fat: 0g
- Cholesterol: 0mg
- Sodium: 300mg
- Carbohydrates: 14g
- Dietary Fiber: 3g
- Sugars: 8g
- Protein: 12g

DIRECTIONS

- turning occasionally, until tofu is browned and vegetables are tender.
- Remove from heat and serve immediately.

GRILLED HALIBUT WITH CITRUS MARINADE

 **Prep Time**
10 Mins

Cook Time
10 Mins

 **Yields**
4 Servings

Marinating Time: 30 Minutes

INGREDIENTS

- 4 halibut fillets (about 6 oz each)
- 2 cloves garlic, minced
- Zest of 1 lemon
- Zest of 1 lime
- Zest of 1 orange
- Juice of 1 lemon
- Juice of 1 lime
- Juice of 1 orange
- 1 tablespoon fresh parsley, chopped
- Salt and pepper to taste

DIRECTIONS

- In a small bowl, mix together the minced garlic, lemon zest, lime zest, orange zest, lemon juice, lime juice, orange juice, parsley, salt, and pepper.
- Place the halibut fillets in a shallow dish or a resealable plastic bag and pour the citrus marinade over them. Make sure the fillets are well coated. Let them marinate in the refrigerator for at least 30 minutes, turning occasionally.
- Preheat your grill to medium-high heat.
- Remove the halibut fillets from the marinade and discard the excess marinade.

NUTRITIONAL FACTS (PER SERVING)

- Calories: 180
- Total Fat: 3g
- Saturated Fat: 0.5g
- Cholesterol: 60mg
- Sodium: 100mg
- Carbohydrates: 5g
- Dietary Fiber: 1g
- Sugars: 2g
- Protein: 34g

DIRECTIONS

- Grill the halibut fillets for about 4-5 minutes per side, or until they are cooked through and easily flake with a fork.
- Serve the grilled halibut hot, garnished with additional fresh parsley if desired.

GREEK STYLE GRILLED LAMB CHOPS

 **Prep Time**
10 Mins

Cook Time
10 Mins

 **Yields**
4 Servings

INGREDIENTS

- 8 lamb loin chops
- 4 cloves garlic, minced
- 2 tablespoons lemon juice
- 2 tablespoons olive oil
- 1 teaspoon dried oregano
- 1 teaspoon dried thyme
- Salt and pepper to taste
- Lemon wedges, for serving
- Chopped fresh parsley, for garnish (optional)

DIRECTIONS

- In a small bowl, mix together the minced garlic, lemon juice, olive oil, dried oregano, dried thyme, salt, and pepper to make the marinade.
- Place the lamb chops in a shallow dish and pour the marinade over them. Make sure each chop is evenly coated. Cover the dish and refrigerate for at least 1 hour, or overnight for best results.
- Preheat your grill to medium-high heat.
- Remove the lamb chops from the marinade and discard any excess marinade.
- Place the lamb chops on the preheated grill and cook for about 4-5 minutes per side for medium-rare,

**NUTRITIONAL FACTS
(PER SERVING)**

- Calories: 300kcal
- Protein: 30g
- Fat: 18g
- Carbohydrates: 2g
- Fiber: 0.5g

DIRECTIONS

- or longer according to your preference.
- Once cooked to your liking, remove the lamb chops from the grill and let them rest for a few minutes before serving.
- Serve the grilled lamb chops with lemon wedges on the side for squeezing over the meat. Garnish with chopped fresh parsley if desired.

MOROCCAN SPICED GRILLED EGGPLANT

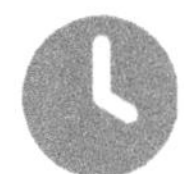 **Prep Time**
10 Mins

Cook Time
10 Mins

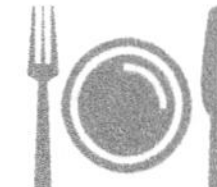 **Yields**
4 Servings

INGREDIENTS

- 2 medium eggplants, sliced into 1/2-inch rounds
- 2 tablespoons olive oil
- 2 cloves garlic, minced
- 1 teaspoon ground cumin
- 1 teaspoon ground coriander
- 1/2 teaspoon smoked paprika
- 1/2 teaspoon ground cinnamon
- Salt and pepper to taste
- Fresh chopped parsley, for garnish

DIRECTIONS

- Preheat your Gas griddle over medium-high heat.
- In a small bowl, mix together the olive oil, minced garlic, ground cumin, ground coriander, smoked paprika, and ground cinnamon to make the spice mixture.
- Brush both sides of the eggplant slices with the spice mixture.
- Place the seasoned eggplant slices on the preheated griddle and cook for about 4-5 minutes on each side, or until tender and grill marks appear.
- Once cooked, remove the eggplant slices from the griddle and place them on a serving platter.
- Garnish with fresh chopped parsley before serving.

**NUTRITIONAL FACTS
(PER SERVING)**

- Calories: 102kcal
- Total Fat: 7g
- Saturated Fat: 1g
- Cholesterol: 0mg
- Sodium: 4mg
- Carbohydrates: 11g
- Dietary Fiber: 5g
- Sugars: 6g
- Protein: 2g

GRIDDLED CHIPOTLE LIME SHRIMP TACOS

Prep Time
20 Mins

Cook Time
8 Mins

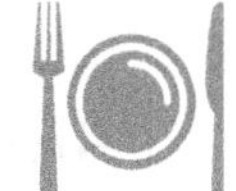

Yields
8 Servings

INGREDIENTS

- 1 pound medium shrimp, peeled and deveined
- 2 tablespoons olive oil
- 2 chipotle peppers in adobo sauce, minced
- 2 cloves garlic, minced
- 2 limes, juiced
- 1 teaspoon ground cumin
- Salt and pepper to taste
- 8 small corn tortillas
- 1 cup shredded cabbage
- 1 avocado, sliced
- Fresh cilantro, for garnish
- Lime wedges, for serving

DIRECTIONS

- In a bowl, combine the olive oil, minced chipotle peppers, minced garlic, lime juice, ground cumin, salt, and pepper. Add the shrimp to the bowl and toss to coat. Let marinate for about 15-20 minutes.
- Preheat your Gas griddle over medium-high heat. Once hot, add the marinated shrimp to the griddle in a single layer.
- Cook the shrimp for 2-3 minutes on each side, or until they are pink and opaque.
- While the shrimp are cooking, warm the corn tortillas on the griddle for about 30 seconds on each side.

NUTRITIONAL FACTS (PER SERVING)

- Calories: 280kcal
- Total Fat: 12g
- Saturated Fat: 1.5g
- Cholesterol: 145mg
- Sodium: 320mg
- Carbohydrates: 25g
- Dietary Fiber: 6g
- Sugars: 2g
- Protein: 20g

DIRECTIONS

- Once the shrimp are cooked, assemble the tacos by placing some shredded cabbage on each tortilla, followed by a few shrimp, sliced avocado, and fresh cilantro.
- Serve the tacos with lime wedges on the side for squeezing over the top.

GRILLED BUFFALO CAULIFLOWER BITES

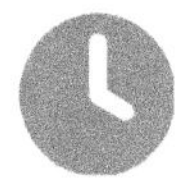 **Prep Time**
10 Mins

Cook Time
20 Mins

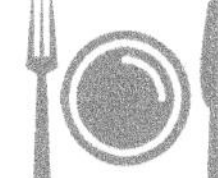 **Yields**
4 Servings

INGREDIENTS

- 1 large head cauliflower, cut into bite-sized florets
- 1/2 cup hot sauce (such as Frank's RedHot)
- 2 tablespoons olive oil
- 1 teaspoon garlic powder
- Salt and pepper to taste
- Optional: Ranch or blue cheese dressing for dipping

DIRECTIONS

- Preheat your gas griddle to medium-high heat.
- In a large bowl, mix together the hot sauce, olive oil, garlic powder, salt, and pepper.
- Add the cauliflower florets to the bowl and toss until evenly coated with the sauce mixture.
- Once the griddle is hot, spread the cauliflower florets in a single layer on the griddle.
- Grill the cauliflower for about 10 minutes, flipping occasionally, until they are tender and charred in spots.
- Remove the cauliflower from the griddle and serve hot with ranch or blue cheese dressing for dipping, if desired.

**NUTRITIONAL FACTS
(PER SERVING)**

- Calories: 100kcal
- Total Fat: 7g
- Saturated Fat: 1g
- Cholesterol: 0mg
- Sodium: 900mg
- Carbohydrates: 8g
- Dietary Fiber: 4g
- Sugars: 2g
- Protein: 3g

GRIDDLED SWEET POTATO HASH BROWNS

 **Prep Time**
10 Mins

Cook Time
14 Mins

 **Yields**
4 Servings

INGREDIENTS

- 2 medium sweet potatoes, peeled and grated
- 1 small onion, finely chopped
- 2 cloves garlic, minced
- 2 tablespoons olive oil
- Salt and pepper to taste
- Optional: chopped fresh herbs such as parsley or chives

DIRECTIONS

- Preheat your Zero Point WW Gas griddle to medium-high heat.
- In a large mixing bowl, combine the grated sweet potatoes, chopped onion, minced garlic, olive oil, salt, and pepper. Mix well until everything is evenly coated.
- Divide the mixture into equal portions and form them into patties, pressing firmly to compact.
- Once the griddle is hot, lightly oil the surface if necessary to prevent sticking.
- Place the sweet potato patties onto the griddle and cook for about 5-7 minutes on each side, or until golden brown and crispy.

NUTRITIONAL FACTS (PER SERVING)

- Calories: 150kcal
- Total Fat: 7g
- Saturated Fat: 1g
- Carbohydrates: 22g
- Dietary Fiber: 4g
- Sugars: 7g
- Protein: 3g

DIRECTIONS

- Serve the sweet potato hash browns hot, garnished with chopped fresh herbs if desired.

GRILLED ASPARAGUS WITH LEMON DILL SAUCE

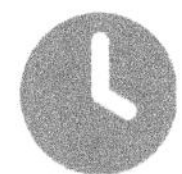 **Prep Time**
10 Mins

Cook Time
7 Mins

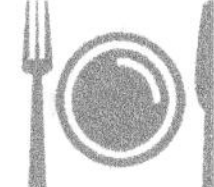 **Yields**
4 Servings

INGREDIENTS

- 1 bunch asparagus, trimmed
- Olive oil spray
- Salt and pepper to taste
- For the Lemon Dill Sauce:
- 1/4 cup fat-free Greek yogurt
- 1 tablespoon fresh dill, chopped
- 1 tablespoon lemon juice
- Zest of 1 lemon
- Salt and pepper to taste

DIRECTIONS

- Preheat your Gas griddle over medium heat.
- Spray the asparagus with olive oil and season with salt and pepper.
- Place the asparagus on the griddle and grill for 5-7 minutes, turning occasionally until tender and slightly charred.
- While the asparagus is grilling, prepare the Lemon Dill Sauce by mixing together the Greek yogurt, fresh dill, lemon juice, lemon zest, salt, and pepper in a small bowl. Set aside.
- Once the asparagus is cooked, remove from the griddle and arrange on a serving platter.
- Drizzle the Lemon Dill Sauce over the grilled asparagus.
- Serve hot and enjoy!

NUTRITIONAL FACTS (PER SERVING)

- Calories: 35kcal
- Total Fat: 0.3g
- Saturated Fat: 0.1g
- Cholesterol: 0mg
- Sodium: 41mg
- Carbohydrates: 5.7g
- Dietary Fiber: 2.5g
- Sugars: 2.4g
- Protein: 3.6g

HONEY GARLIC GLAZED GRILLED TOFU

Prep Time
15 Mins

Cook Time
15 Mins

Yields
4 Servings

INGREDIENTS

- 14 oz extra firm tofu, drained and pressed
- 2 tablespoons soy sauce (low sodium if preferred)
- 2 tablespoons honey (or maple syrup for a vegan option)
- 2 cloves garlic, minced
- 1 tablespoon rice vinegar
- 1 tablespoon sesame oil
- 1 tablespoon grated fresh ginger
- Salt and pepper to taste
- Cooking spray (or oil for greasing the grill)

DIRECTIONS

- Drain the tofu and press it to remove excess moisture. You can do this by wrapping it in a clean kitchen towel and placing something heavy on top (like a cast-iron skillet or a few heavy books) for about 15-20 minutes.
- In a small bowl, whisk together soy sauce, honey (or maple syrup), minced garlic, rice vinegar, sesame oil, grated ginger, salt, and pepper.
- Once pressed, slice the tofu into ½-inch thick slices. Place them in a shallow dish or a resealable plastic bag. Pour the marinade over the tofu, ensuring all slices are coated.

NUTRITIONAL FACTS (PER SERVING)

- Calories: 170kcal
- Protein: 12g
- Fat: 8g
- Carbohydrates: 15g
- Fiber: 1g

DIRECTIONS

- Marinate for at least 30 minutes, or ideally for a few hours in the refrigerator, flipping the tofu halfway through if using a dish.
- Preheat your grill to medium-high heat. If using an indoor grill pan, heat it over medium-high heat on the stovetop.
- Lightly grease the grill grates with cooking spray or oil. Place the marinated tofu slices on the grill and cook for about 5-7 minutes on each side, or until grill marks form and the tofu is heated through.
- During the last few minutes of grilling, brush the tofu slices with any remaining marinade to create a glaze. Be careful not to let the glaze burn.
- Once the tofu is nicely grilled and glazed, remove it from the grill and serve immediately.

GRIDDLED GREEK HALLOUMI CHEESE

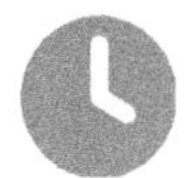 **Prep Time**
10 Mins

Cook Time
5 Mins

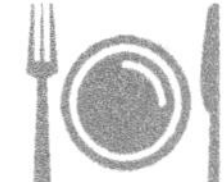 **Yields**
4 Servings

INGREDIENTS

- 1 block of halloumi cheese
- 1 tablespoon olive oil
- 1 teaspoon dried oregano
- 1 teaspoon dried thyme
- 1 teaspoon dried rosemary
- 1 lemon, cut into wedges (for serving)
- Freshly ground black pepper, to taste

DIRECTIONS

- Slice the halloumi cheese into 1/4-inch thick slices.
- In a small bowl, mix together the olive oil, dried oregano, dried thyme, and dried rosemary.
- Preheat your Gas griddle over medium-high heat.
- Brush the herb-infused olive oil mixture onto both sides of the halloumi slices.
- Place the halloumi slices on the preheated griddle and cook for 2-3 minutes on each side, or until golden brown and crispy.
- Once cooked, remove the halloumi slices from the griddle and place them on a serving platter.

NUTRITIONAL FACTS (PER SERVING)

- Calories: 180kcal
- Total Fat: 14g
- Saturated Fat: 8g
- Cholesterol: 30mg
- Sodium: 500mg
- Total Carbohydrates: 1g
- Dietary Fiber: 0g
- Sugars: 0g
- Protein: 12g

DIRECTIONS

- Serve the griddled halloumi cheese hot with lemon wedges on the side for squeezing over the top.
- Garnish with freshly ground black pepper to taste.
- Enjoy your delicious Griddled Greek Halloumi Cheese!

GRILLED CHIMICHURRI STEAK

 **Prep Time**
10 Mins

Cook Time
10 Mins

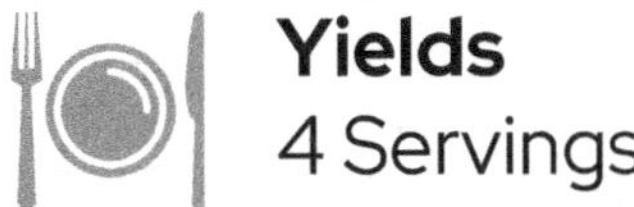 **Yields**
4 Servings

INGREDIENTS

- 4 (6 oz each) lean beef steaks (such as sirloin or flank)
- Salt and pepper to taste
- For the chimichurri sauce:
- 1 cup fresh parsley, chopped
- 1/4 cup fresh cilantro, chopped
- 3 cloves garlic, minced
- 1/4 cup red wine vinegar
- 1/2 cup olive oil
- 1 teaspoon dried oregano
- 1/2 teaspoon red pepper flakes (adjust to taste)
- Salt and pepper to taste

DIRECTIONS

- Preheat your gas griddle to medium-high heat.
- Season the steaks generously with salt and pepper on both sides.
- In a bowl, mix together all the ingredients for the chimichurri sauce.
- Place the steaks on the hot griddle and cook for about 4-5 minutes on each side for medium-rare, or adjust the cooking time according to your preference.
- Once the steaks are cooked to your liking, remove them from the griddle and let them rest for a few minutes.
- Serve the steaks topped with chimichurri sauce. You can also serve with a side of vegetables or salad.

NUTRITIONAL FACTS (PER SERVING)

- Calories: 350kcal
- Total Fat: 25g
- Saturated Fat: 6g
- Cholesterol: 90mg
- Sodium: 80mg
- Carbohydrates: 2g
- Dietary Fiber: 1g
- Sugars: 0g
- Protein: 29g

GRILLED RATATOUILLE FLATBREAD PIZZA

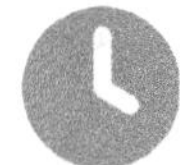

Prep Time
15 Mins

Cook Time
20 Mins

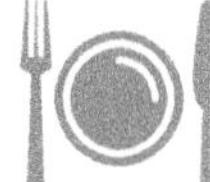

Yields
4 Servings

INGREDIENTS

- 1 medium eggplant, thinly sliced
- 1 medium zucchini, thinly sliced
- 1 red bell pepper, sliced
- 1 yellow bell pepper, sliced
- 1 red onion, thinly sliced
- 2 cloves garlic, minced
- 2 tablespoons olive oil
- Salt and pepper to taste
- 4 flatbreads or naan breads
- 1 cup marinara sauce
- 2 cups shredded mozzarella cheese
- Fresh basil leaves for garnish (optional)

DIRECTIONS

- Preheat your gas griddle to medium-high heat.
- In a large bowl, toss the eggplant, zucchini, bell peppers, onion, and garlic with olive oil, salt, and pepper.
- Grill the sliced vegetables on the preheated griddle until they are tender and have grill marks, about 5-7 minutes per side. Remove from the griddle and set aside.
- Place the flatbreads on the griddle and spread each with marinara sauce.
- Top each flatbread with grilled vegetables and sprinkle with shredded mozzarella cheese.
- Close the lid of the griddle and cook for 5-7 minutes, or until the cheese is melted and bubbly.

NUTRITIONAL FACTS (PER SERVING)

- Calories: 380kcal
- Total Fat: 18g
- Saturated Fat: 7g
- Trans Fat: 0g
- Cholesterol: 25mg
- Sodium: 720mg
- Total Carbohydrates: 41g
- Dietary Fiber: 5g
- Sugars: 8g
- Protein: 16g

DIRECTIONS

- Remove the pizzas from the griddle and garnish with fresh basil leaves if desired.
- Slice and serve hot.

GRILLED BRUSCHETTA CHICKEN

 **Prep Time**
10 Mins

Cook Time
15 Mins

 **Yields**
4 Servings

INGREDIENTS

- 4 boneless, skinless chicken breasts
- 2 cups cherry tomatoes, halved
- 2 cloves garlic, minced
- 1/4 cup fresh basil leaves, chopped
- 1 tablespoon balsamic vinegar
- 1 tablespoon olive oil
- Salt and pepper to taste

DIRECTIONS

- In a bowl, combine the cherry tomatoes, garlic, basil, balsamic vinegar, olive oil, salt, and pepper. Mix well and set aside to marinate while you prepare the chicken.
- Preheat your gas griddle over medium-high heat.
- Season the chicken breasts with salt and pepper.
- Place the chicken breasts on the preheated griddle and cook for about 6-8 minutes per side, or until cooked through and no longer pink in the center.
- While the chicken is cooking, grill the marinated cherry tomato mixture on the griddle for about 4-5 minutes, or until the tomatoes are slightly softened and charred.

NUTRITIONAL FACTS (PER SERVING)

- Calories: 200kcal
- Protein: 25g
- Carbohydrates: 5g
- Fat: 7g
- Fiber: 1g

DIRECTIONS

- Once the chicken is cooked through, remove it from the griddle and let it rest for a few minutes.
- Serve the grilled chicken topped with the grilled bruschetta mixture.

GRIDDLED CAULIFLOWER STEAKS WITH TAHINI SAUCE

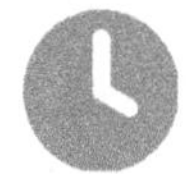 **Prep Time**
10 Mins

Cook Time
20 Mins

 **Yields**
4 Servings

INGREDIENTS

- 1 large head cauliflower
- Salt and pepper to taste
- 2 tablespoons olive oil

For the tahini sauce:

- 1/4 cup tahini
- 2 tablespoons lemon juice
- 2 tablespoons water
- 1 clove garlic, minced
- Salt to taste
- Optional: chopped parsley for garnish

DIRECTIONS

- Preheat your gas griddle to medium-high heat.
- Remove the leaves from the cauliflower and trim the stem end to create a flat base.
- Slice the cauliflower into 1-inch thick steaks, keeping the core intact to hold the steaks together.
- Brush both sides of each cauliflower steak with olive oil and season with salt and pepper.
- Place the cauliflower steaks on the preheated griddle and cook for about 8-10 minutes on each side, or until tender and grill marks appear.
- While the cauliflower is grilling, prepare the tahini sauce. In a small bowl, whisk together tahini, lemon juice, water,

- Calories: 150kcal
- Total Fat: 12g
- Saturated Fat: 1.5g
- Sodium: 120mg
- Total Carbohydrates: 8g
- Dietary Fiber: 3g
- Sugars: 2g
- Protein: 4g

DIRECTIONS

- minced garlic, and salt until smooth and creamy. If the sauce is too thick, you can add more water to reach your desired consistency.
- Once the cauliflower steaks are cooked, transfer them to a serving plate and drizzle with tahini sauce.
- Garnish with chopped parsley if desired, and serve hot.

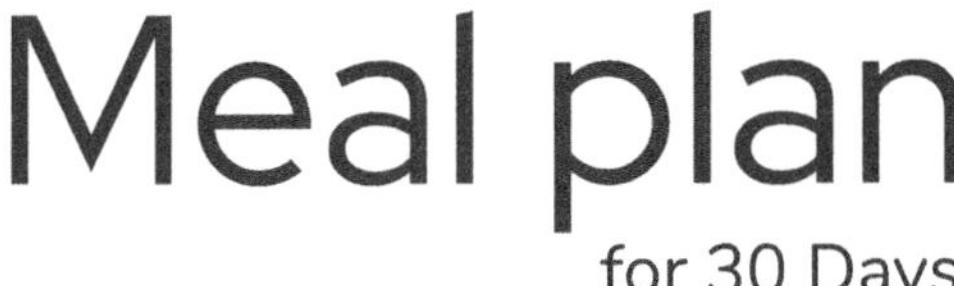

Meal plan

for 30 Days

Dates
____

	BREAKFAST	LUNCH	DINNER
MON	Scrambled eggs with spinach and tomatoes	Grilled chicken breast with a mixed green salad (lettuce, cucumber, bell peppers) and balsamic vinaigrette	Baked salmon with steamed broccoli and cauliflower
TUE	Greek yogurt with fresh berries and a sprinkle of chia seeds	Turkey lettuce wraps with hummus and sliced veggies	Stir-fried shrimp with bell peppers, onions, and zucchini served over cauliflower rice
WED	Oatmeal topped with sliced banana and a dollop of almond butter	Quinoa salad with cherry tomatoes, cucumber, red onion, and lemon-tahini dressing	Grilled tofu with roasted Brussels sprouts and carrots
THU	Veggie omelet (with mushrooms, onions, bell peppers) cooked in olive oil	Lentil soup with a side of mixed greens dressed with lemon juice	Baked cod with asparagus and a side of mixed bean salad
FRI	Smoothie made with spinach, frozen berries, banana, and almond milk	Grilled shrimp skewers with a side of Greek salad (tomatoes, cucumbers, olives, feta cheese)	Zucchini noodles with marinara sauce and grilled chicken breast
SAT	Cottage cheese topped with pineapple chunks and a sprinkle of cinnamon	Tuna salad lettuce wraps with diced celery and carrots	Turkey chili with black beans, diced tomatoes, and bell peppers

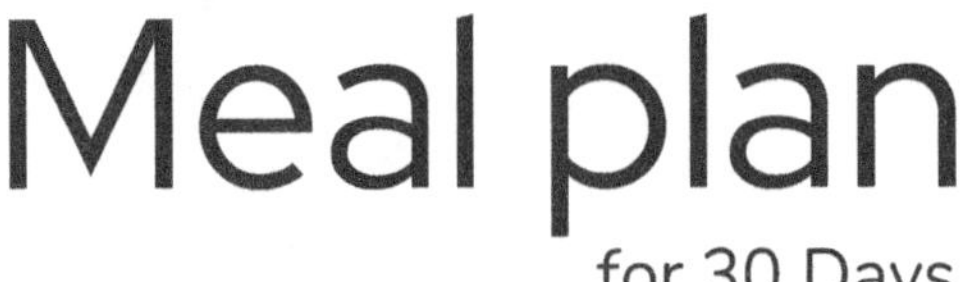

Meal plan
for 30 Days

Dates

____

	BREAKFAST	LUNCH	DINNER
SUN	Whole grain toast with mashed avocado and sliced tomato	Egg salad stuffed in bell pepper halves served with a side of carrot sticks	Grilled steak with roasted green beans and a side of quinoa

Week 2-4

- Continue to repeat and vary these meal ideas throughout the 30-day period, incorporating a wide range of fruits, vegetables, lean proteins, and whole grains. Remember to drink plenty of water throughout the day and listen to your body's hunger and fullness cues.

ZERO POINT FOOD LIST

Zero Point Fruits

- Apples
- Apricots
- Bananas
- Blackberries
- Blueberries
- Cantaloupe
- Cherries
- Clementine
- Coconut
- Cranberries
- Dates
- Dragon Fruit
- Figs
- Grapefruit
- Grapes (any variety)
- Guava
- Honeydew Melon
- Jackfruit
- Kiwi
- Lemon
- Lime
- Mango
- Oranges
- Passion Fruit
- Peach
- Pears
- Pineapple
- Plums
- Pomegranates
- Raspberries
- Starfruit
- Strawberries
- Watermelon

BEANS & LEGUMES

- Adzuki beans
- Alfalfa sprouts
- Bean sprouts
- Black beans
- Black-eyed peas
- Cannellini beans
- Chickpeas
- Edamame
- Fava beans
- Great Northern beans
- Hominy
- Kidney beans
- Lentils
- Lima beans
- Lupini beans
- Navy beans
- Pinto beans
- Refried beans, canned, fat-free
- Soy beans

CHICKEN & TURKEY BREAST

- Ground chicken breast
- Ground turkey, 98% fat-free
- Ground turkey breast
- Skinless chicken breast
- Skinless turkey breast

EGGS

- Egg substitute
- Egg whites
- Egg yolks
- Eggs

Zero Point Vegetables (Starchy & Non-Starchy)

- Arrowroot, raw
- Artichoke
- Arugula
- Asparagus
- Broccoli
- Beans (black, adzuki, cannellini, garbanzo, kidney, great northern, lima, pinto, etc.)
- Beans, refried (canned, fat-free, no added sugar)
- Green Beans
- Bok Choy
- Brussel Sprouts
- Cabbage
- Carrots
- Cauliflower
- Celery
- Chard
- Chickpeas
- Collards
- Corn
- Cucumber
- Daikon
- Edamame
- Eggplant
- Endive
- Fennel
- Ginger Root
- Kale
- Leeks
- Lettuce (any variety)
- Mushrooms
- Okra
- Peas
- Peppers (bell)
- Pickles (without sugar)
- Pumpkin
- Radishes
- Scallions (green onions)
- Spinach
- Sprouts
- Squash
- Tomatoes
- Turnips
- Zucchini

Zero Point Herbs and Spices

- Basil
- Chives
- Cinnamon
- Dill Weed
- Garlic
- Garlic Salt
- Italian Seasoning
- Oregano
- Paprika
- Parsley
- Pepper
- Peppermint
- Pumpkin Spice
- Rosemary
- Sage
- Salt
- Thyme

Zero Point Meat, Seafood and Poultry

- Calamari, grilled
- Chicken Breast (boneless, skinless)
- Crab (Alasaka king, Dungeness, queen, king)
- Crayfish
- Eggs
- Bass Fish
- Bluefish
- Carp
- Catfish
- Cod
- Eel
- Grouper
- Haddock
- Halibut
- Lobster
- Mackerel Fish
- Mussels
- Octopus
- Oysters
- Salmon (Atlantic and farm raised)
- Sardines
- Sea Bass
- Shrimp
- Sturgeon Fish
- Swordfish
- Tilapia Fish
- Tuna (canned in water, drained)
- Tofu
- Trout (rainbow)
- Turkey breast (ground, tenderloin, etc. 99% fat-free)

FISH/SHELLFISH

- Abalone
- Alaskan king crab
- Anchovies, in water
- Arctic char
- Bluefish
- Branzino
- Butterfish
- Canned tuna, in water
- Carp
- Catfish
- Caviar
- Clams
- Cod
- Crabmeat, lump
- Crayfish
- Cuttlefish
- Dungeness crab
- Eel
- Fish roe
- Flounder
- Grouper
- Haddock
- Halibut
- Herring
- Lobster
- Mahi mahi
- Monkfish
- Mussels
- Octopus
- Orange roughy
- Oysters
- Perch
- Pike
- Pollock
- Pompano
- Salmon
- Sardines, canned in water or sauce
- Sashimi
- Scallops
- Sea bass
- Sea cucumber
- Sea urchin
- Shrimp
- Smelt
- Smoked haddock
- Smoked salmon
- Smoked sturgeon
- Smoked trout
- Smoked whitefish
- Snails
- Snapper
- Sole
- Squid

- Steelhead trout
- Striped bass
- Sturgeon
- Swordfish
- Tilapia
- Trout
- Tuna
- Turbot
- Wahoo
- Whitefish

Zero Point Drinks

- Water
- Coffee, black (without sugar)
- Coke Zero (all varieties)
- Diet Coke (all varieties)
- Fresca (all varieties)
- Gatorade Zero
- Sparkling Ice Water (all flavors) etc.

- **Zero Point Snacks**
- Applesauce, unsweetened
- Fruit cup (canned in water pack, no sugar added)
- Fruit cup (fresh)
- Vegetable Sticks
- Yogurt (greek, plain, fat-free, unsweetened)

IMPORTANT NOTICE!!!

We chose to make costs low so it can be accessible to everyone who would love to lose weight. As a result, we didn't include pictures for each recipes.

Please, reach out to us at **popoolaadenike805@gmail.com** if you would like to receive the pictures for each recipes.

HAPPY COOKING!

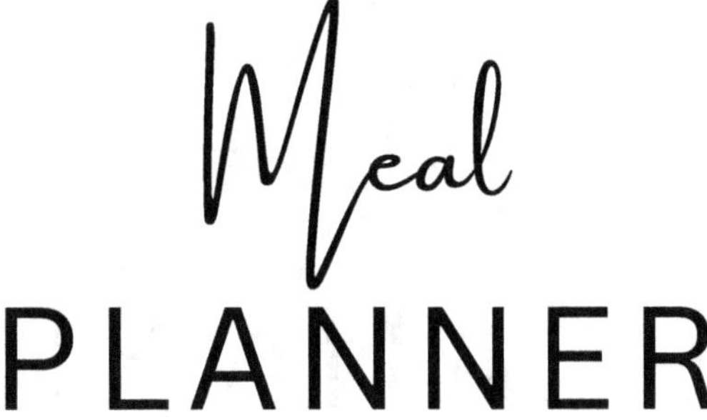

WEEK :

DATE :

MONDAY

B

L

D

S

TUESDAY

B

L

D

S

WEDNESDAY

B

L

D

S

THURSDAY

B

L

D

S

FRIDAY

B

L

D

S

SATURDAY

B

L

D

S

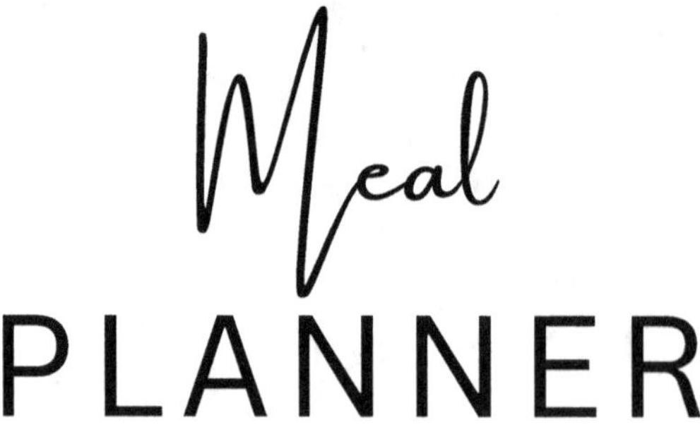

WEEK :

DATE :

MONDAY

B

L

D

S

TUESDAY

B

L

D

S

WEDNESDAY

B

L

D

S

THURSDAY

B

L

D

S

FRIDAY

B

L

D

S

SATURDAY

B

L

D

S

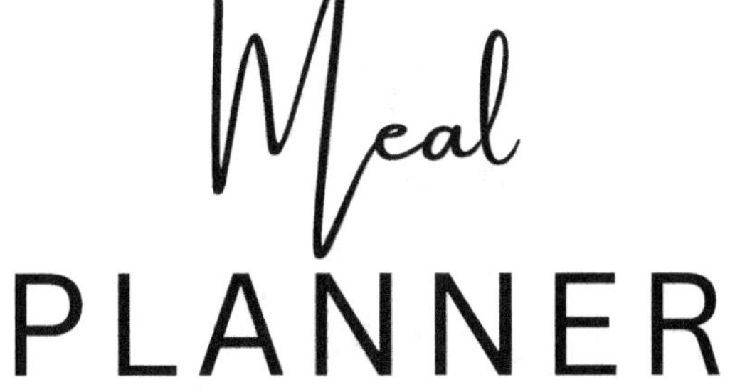

Meal PLANNER

WEEK :

DATE :

MONDAY

B

L

D

S

THURSDAY

B

L

D

S

TUESDAY

B

L

D

S

FRIDAY

B

L

D

S

WEDNESDAY

B

L

D

S

SATURDAY

B

L

D

S

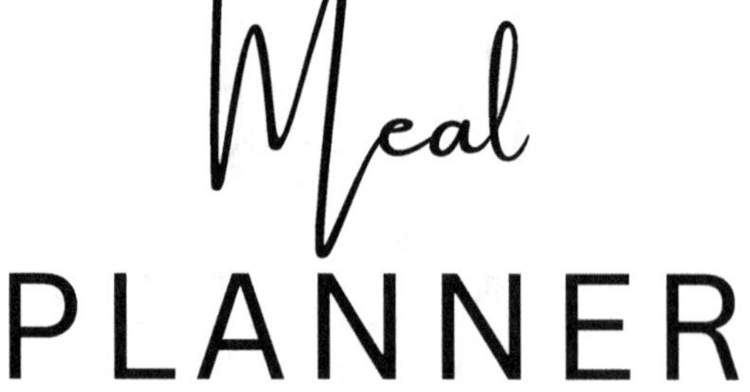

Meal PLANNER

WEEK :

DATE :

MONDAY

B

L

D

S

THURSDAY

B

L

D

S

TUESDAY

B

L

D

S

FRIDAY

B

L

D

S

WEDNESDAY

B

L

D

S

SATURDAY

B

L

D

S

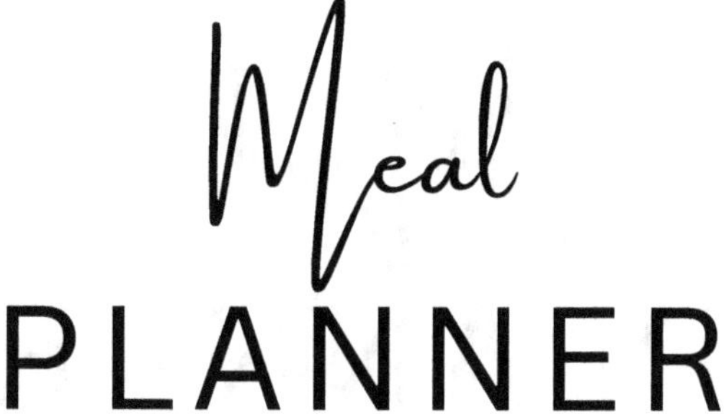

WEEK :

DATE :

MONDAY

B

L

D

S

TUESDAY

B

L

D

S

WEDNESDAY

B

L

D

S

THURSDAY

B

L

D

S

FRIDAY

B

L

D

S

SATURDAY

B

L

D

S

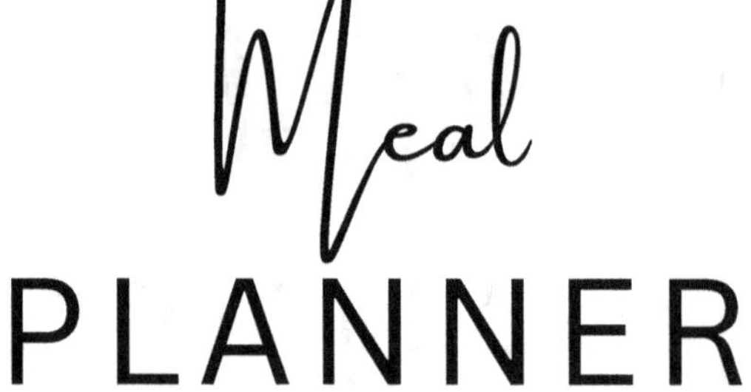

Meal PLANNER

WEEK :

DATE :

MONDAY

B

L

D

S

TUESDAY

B

L

D

S

WEDNESDAY

B

L

D

S

THURSDAY

B

L

D

S

FRIDAY

B

L

D

S

SATURDAY

B

L

D

S

www.ingramcontent.com/pod-product-compliance
Lightning Source LLC
Chambersburg PA
CBHW080728260726
48660CB00010B/3741